- Clinical Nutrition -

BASICS OF ARTIFICIAL NUTRITION

Enteral and Parenteral Nutrition

FIRST EDITION

Dr. Amin Gasmi

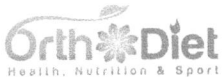

© **Copyright 2020 by Dr. Amin Gasmi - All rights reserved.**

The contents of this book may not be reproduced, duplicated or transmitted without direct written permission from the author.

Under no circumstances will any legal responsibility or blame be held against the publisher for any reparation, damages, or monetary loss due to the information herein, either directly or indirectly.

Legal Notice:

This book is copyright protected. This is only for personal use. You cannot amend, distribute, sell, use, quote or paraphrase any part or the content within this book without the consent of the author.

Disclaimer Notice:

Please note the information contained within this document is for educational and entertainment purposes only. Every attempt has been made to provide accurate, up to date and reliable complete information. No warranties of any kind are expressed or implied. Readers acknowledge that the author is not engaging in the rendering of legal, financial, medical or professional advice. The content of this book has been derived from various sources. Please consult a licensed professional before attempting any techniques outlined in this book.

By reading this document, the reader agrees that under no circumstances is the author responsible for any losses, direct or indirect, which are incurred as a result of the use of information contained within this document, including, but not limited to, —errors, omissions, or inaccuracies.

DEDICATION

To the ultimate power of the universe, the power of love. For me, more than all: dad, mom, my wife, Alain, Cherif and Salva.

ACKNOWLEDGEMENT

I thank all those who throughout my life have contributed to my training and make me what I have become today: God, my family, my teachers, my colleagues, my friends, my students, my patients, my athletes, and everyone I have met on my way. I am also indebted to a large number of books and scientific articles, and I cannot thank their authors enough for their sharing and generosity.

TABLE OF CONTENTS

Dedication iii

Acknowledgement iv

ARTIFICIAL NUTRITION: ENTERAL AND PARENTERAL 1

    Features of Human Metabolism During Fasting 3

    Gastrointestinal Tract During Fasting and in Critical Condition 4

PRINCIPLES OF NUTRITIONAL SUPPORT 7

    Assessment of Energy Needs of The Patient................................... 8

ENTERAL NUTRITION 11

    Enteral Nutrition Benefits 13

    Indications for Enteral Nutrition 13

    Contraindications to Enteral Nutrition... 15

    General Recommendations for Enteral Nutrition 17

    Enteral Nutrition Access Choice 18

    Types of Probes for Enteral Nutrition 20

    Methods of Introducing Nutrient Mixtures into the Probe 21

    When to Start Enteral Nutrition 22

ENTERAL NUTRITION MODES...23

ENTERAL NUTRITION MIXTURES 26

    General Requirements for Enteral Mixtures 26

    Enteral Nutrition Control 28

    Enteral Nutrition Protocol In Intensive Care Units 28

    Enteral Nutrition Complications 29

    Classification Of Enteral Nutrition Complications 30

    Residual Volumes, Vomiting, Regurgitation, And Aspiration 31

    Diarrhea 32

    Bloating 34

    Constipation 35

    Metabolic Complications 35

    Migration, Clogging Of Probes And Tubes 37

    Other Complications 39

    About Sterility With Enteral Nutrition 40

PARENTERAL NUTRITION 41

    Classification Of Parenteral Nutrition 43

    The Main Tasks Of Parenteral Nutrition 43

    Parenteral Nutrition Concepts 44

    Basic Principles Of Parenteral Nutrition 45

    Rules For Parenteral Nutrition 45

    Indications For Parenteral Nutrition 46

    Indications For Parenteral Nutrition 47

    Contraindications For Parenteral Nutrition 48

    Providing Parenteral Nutrition...................................... 49

Preparations For Parenteral Nutrition 51

Characteristics Of Parenteral Nutrition 51

Parenteral Nutrition Components 52

Assessment Of The Patient's Condition If
Parenteral Nutrition Is Necessary 53

The Energy Needs Of The Body 54

Complications Of Parenteral Nutrition 55

Technical Complications 55

METABOLIC COMPLICATIONS 56

Organopathological Complications 56

Septic Complications 57

Complications Associated With The Introduction
Of Fat Emulsions 57

ENTERAL OR PARENTERAL NUTRITION? 59

AUTHOR'S PRESENTATION 61

REFERENCES 62

ARTIFICIAL NUTRITION

Enteral And Parenteral

Artificial nutrition is today one of the basic types of treatment for patients in a hospital. There is practically no field of medicine in which it would not be used. The most relevant is the use of artificial nutrition (or artificial nutritional support) for surgical, gastroenterological, oncological, nephrological, and geriatric contingents of patients.

Nutritional support is a complex therapeutic measure aimed at identifying and correcting violations of the nutritional status of the body using methods of nutritional therapy (enteral and parenteral nutrition). This is the process of providing the body with nutrients using methods other than ordinary meals.

"The doctor's inability to provide nutrition to the patient should be regarded as a decision to starve him to death. A decision for which in most cases it would be difficult to find an excuse." - Arvid Vretlind

Timely and adequate nutritional support can significantly reduce the incidence of infectious complications and mortality of patients, to improve the quality of life of patients and accelerate their rehabilitation.

Artificial nutritional support can be complete when all (or the main part) of the patient's nutritional needs are provided artificially, or partially, if the introduction of nutrients by the enteral and parenteral route is complementary to normal (oral) nutrition.

Indications for artificial nutritional support are diverse. In general, they can be described as any diseases in which the patient's need for nutrients cannot be provided naturally. Usually, these are diseases of the gastrointestinal tract that do not allow the patient to eat adequately. Artificial nutrition may also be necessary for patients with metabolic problems - severe hypermetabolism, catabolism, and high loss of nutrients.

The rule of 7 days or a 7% reduction in body weight is widely known. It means that artificial nutrition must be carried out in cases where the patient for 7 days or more will not be able to eat naturally, or if the patient has lost more than 7% of the recommended body weight.

Assessment of the effectiveness of nutritional support includes the following indicators: dynamics of parameters of nutritional status; state of nitrogen balance; the course of the underlying disease, the state of the surgical wound; general dynamics of the patient's condition, severity and course of organ dysfunction.

There are two main forms of artificial nutritional support: enteral (probe) and parenteral (intravascular) nutrition.

Features of Human Metabolism During Fasting

The primary reaction of the body in response to the cessation of nutrient intake from the outside is the use of glycogen and glycogen depots as an energy source (glycogenolysis). However, the supply of glycogen in the body is usually not large and is depleted during the first two to three days. Subsequently, the body's structural proteins (gluconeogenesis) become the easiest and most affordable source of energy. In the process of gluconeogenesis, glucose-dependent tissues produce ketone bodies, which, according to the feedback reaction, slow down the main metabolism and the oxidation of lipid reserves as an energy source begins. Gradually, the body goes into a protein-saving mode of functioning, and gluconeogenesis resumes only with complete depletion of fat stores. So, if in the first days of fasting, protein loss is 10-12g per day, the loss of proteins will be accelerated and the protein deficiency will appear rapidly.

In critically ill patients, a powerful release of stress hormones occurs - catecholamines, glucagon, which have a pronounced catabolic effect. In this case, production is disrupted, or the response to such hormones with anabolic action as growth hormone and insulin is blocked. As often happens in critical conditions, an adaptive reaction aimed at breaking down proteins and providing the body with substrates for building new tissues and healing wounds gets out of control and becomes purely destructive. Due to catecholaminemia, the body's transition to the use of fat as an energy source slows down. In this case (with severe fever, polytrauma, burns), up to 300 g of structural protein per day can burn. This condition was called autocaniballism. Energy costs increase by 50-150%.

The fundamental difference between physiological adaptation to starvation and adaptive reactions in terminal states is that in the first case, an adaptive decrease in energy demand is noted, and in the second, energy consumption increases significantly. Therefore, in post-aggressive states, negative nitrogen balance should be avoided since protein depletion ultimately leads to death, which occurs when more than 30% of the total nitrogen of the body is lost.

Gastrointestinal Tract During Fasting and in Critical Condition

In critical conditions of the body, conditions often arise under which adequate perfusion and oxygenation of the gastrointestinal tract are impaired. This leads to damage to the cells of the intestinal epithelium with an impaired barrier function. Violations are aggravated if, for a long time, there are no nutrients in the lumen of the gastrointestinal tract (during starvation), since the cells of the mucosa receive nutrition largely directly from the chyme.

An important damage to the digestive tract is any centralization of blood circulation. With the centralization of blood circulation, perfusion of the intestine and parenchymal organs decreases. In critical conditions, this is compounded by the frequent use of adrenomimetic drugs to maintain systemic hemodynamics. In time, the restoration of normal intestinal perfusion lags behind the restoration of normal perfusion of vital organs. The absence of chyme in the intestinal lumen disrupts the entry of antioxidants and their precursors into enterocytes and exacerbates reperfusion lesions. Due to autoregulatory mechanisms, the liver suffers slightly less from a decrease in blood flow, but its perfusion decreases.

When fasting, microbial translocation develops, that is, the penetration of microorganisms from the lumen of the gastrointestinal tract through the mucous barrier into the blood or lymph flow. Escherichia coli, Enterococcus, and Candida bacteria are mainly involved in translocation. In certain amounts, microbial translocation is always present. The bacteria penetrating the submucosal layer are captured by macrophages and transported to the systemic lymph nodes. When they enter the bloodstream, they are captured and destroyed by the Kupffer cells of the liver. Stable equilibrium is disturbed with uncontrolled growth of intestinal microflora and a change in its normal composition (i.e., with the development of dysbiosis), impaired mucosal permeability, and impaired local intestinal immunity. It is proved that microbial translocation occurs in critical patients. It intensifies in the presence of risk factors (burns and severe trauma, broad-spectrum systemic antibiotics, pancreatitis, hemorrhagic shock, reperfusion lesions, exclusion of solid foods, etc.), and it is often the cause of infectious lesions in critical patients. In the USA, 10% of hospitalized patients develop a nosocomial infection. This is 2 million people, 580 thousand deaths, and treatment costs of about 4.5 billion dollars.

Disorders of the intestinal barrier function, expressed in mucosal atrophy and impaired permeability, in critical patients develop quite early and are already apparent on the 4th day of fasting. Many studies have shown the beneficial effect of early enteral nutrition (the first 6 hours from admission) to prevent mucosal atrophy.

In the absence of enteral nutrition, not only atrophy of the intestinal mucosa occurs, but also atrophy of the so-called intestinal lymphoid tissue (gut-associated lymphoid tissue - GALT). These are Peyer's patches, mesenteric lymph nodes, lymphocytes of the epithelium, and the basement membrane. Maintaining proper nutrition through the intestines helps to maintain the immunity of the whole organism in a normal state.

PRINCIPLES OF NUTRITIONAL SUPPORT

One of the founders of the doctrine of artificial nutrition, Arvid Wretlind, formulated the principles of nutritional support:

- **Timeliness**

  Artificial nutrition should be started as early as possible, even before the development of nutritional disorders. You cannot wait for the development of protein-energy deficiency since cachexia is much easier to prevent than to treat.

- **Optimality**

  Artificial nutrition must be carried out until the nutritional status is stabilized.

- **Adequacy**

  Nutrition should cover the energy needs of the body and be balanced in the composition of nutrients and meet the needs of the patient in them.

Assessment of Energy Needs of The Patient

When conducting nutritional support (enterol and parenteral nutrition), it is necessary to assess the patient's energy needs correctly. Assessment of the energy needs of a critical patient can be carried out by calculation methods or using indirect calorimetry.

It is easiest to evaluate the initial energy requirement for a critical patient as 25 to 35 non-protein calories per kg of body weight per day. Energy costs are usually in the range of 1500-3000 kcal.

More precise and complex calculation formulas exist, such as the Harris-Benedict equation.

The equation includes the height, weight, age, and gender of the patient with the addition of the so-called stress factor:

$$EOO \text{ (men)} = 66 + (13.7 \times W) + (5 \times H) - (6.8 \times A)$$

$$EOO \text{ (women)} = 655 + (9.9 \times W) + (1.8 \times H) - (4.7 \times A)$$

Where EOO - the main exchange (kcal)

W - body weight (kg)

H - height (cm)

A - age (years)

Surgical intervention can add up to 10%, severe trauma up to 30%, sepsis from 20 to 50% and severe burns up to 100% to the calculated values.

On average, the calculation methods quite accurately correspond to the real energy consumption, but in each case, the fluctuations can be from 30 to + 50%, and you can never accurately predict whether the energy demand of this particular patient will be higher or lower than the calculated level. Thus, a deviation of 20-30% in calculations in critical patients is permissible.

For various conditions, energy demand is calculated by multiplying the basal metabolic rate by various factors:

- The state of rest on the bed is 1.2

- Outpatient conditions - 1.3

- Anabolic conditions - 1.5

In stressful situations, the intensity of energy consumption changes, and depending on the patient's condition, the daily energy requirement may be as follows:

- After planned abdominal operations - 30-40 kcal/kg.

- After radical surgery for cancer - 50-60 kcal/kg.

- In severe mechanical skeletal injuries - 50-70 kcal/kg.

- With traumatic brain injuries - 60-80 kcal/kg.

A more accurate assessment of energy requirements is carried out for each patient by indirect calorimetry in conditions of basic metabolism (for oxygen consumption and carbon dioxide emissions). There are special units for ventilators, allowing these measurements. Since maintaining the parameters of the basal metabolism during the whole day can be difficult, studies have recently appeared showing the possibility of measurement within 30 minutes to 2 hours. They quite accurately predict daily parameters if the study is carried out between 11 and 15 hours and with blood pressure, heart rate, and BH parameters close to the average daily values.

ENTERAL NUTRITION 3

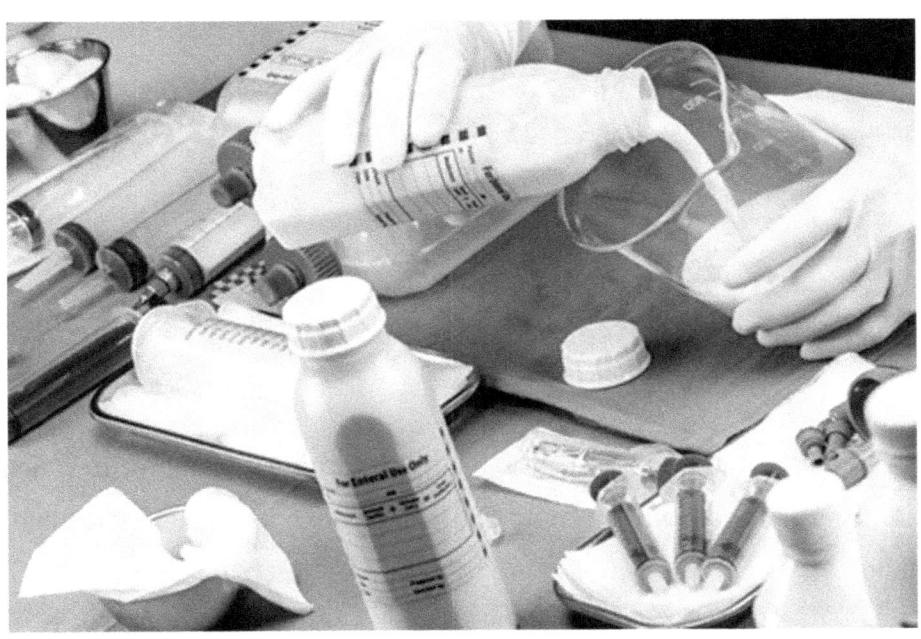

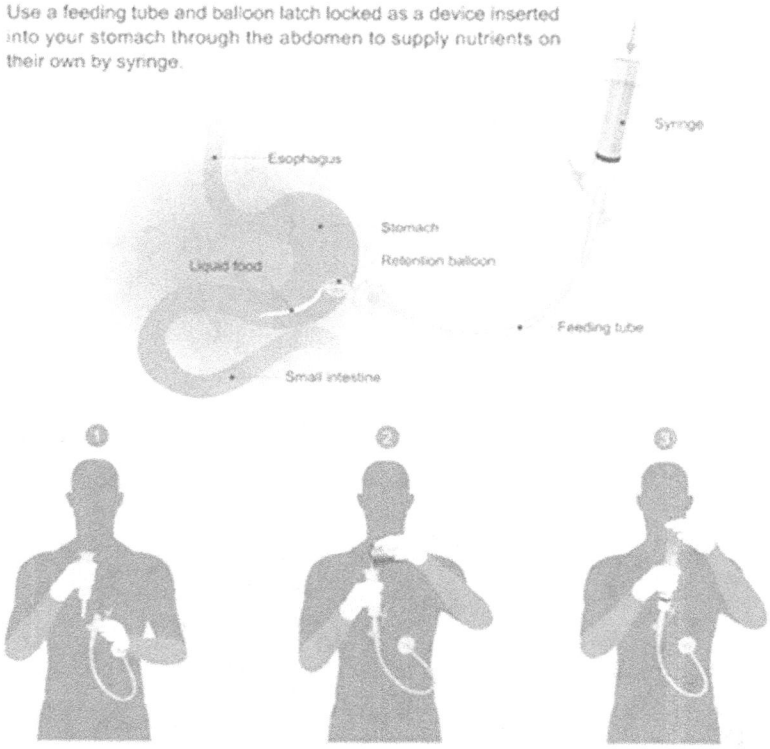

E nteral nutrition (EP) is a type of nutritional therapy in which nutrients are administered orally or through a stomach (intestinal) tube.

Enteral nutrition refers to types of artificial nutrition and, therefore, is not carried out through natural routes. For enteral nutrition, this or that access is necessary, as well as special devices for the introduction of nutritional mixtures.

Some authors refer to enteral nutrition as the only method that bypasses the oral cavity. Others include oral nutrition in mixtures other than regular foods. In this case, two main options are distinguished: probe nutrition - the introduction of enteral mixtures into the probe or stoma, and "sipping" (sipping, sip feeding) - oral administration of a special mixture for enteral nutrition in small sips (usually through a tube).

Enteral Nutrition Benefits

Enteral nutrition has several advantages over parenteral nutrition:

- Enteral nutrition is more physiological.
- Enteral nutrition is more economical.
- Enteral nutrition practically does not cause life-threatening complications and does not require compliance with strict sterility conditions.
- Enteral nutrition makes it possible to provide the body with the necessary substrates to a greater extent.
- Enteral nutrition prevents the development of atrophic processes in the gastrointestinal tract.

Indications for Enteral Nutrition

Indications for EP are almost all situations when a patient with a functioning gastrointestinal tract can't meet protein and energy requirements in the usual, oral way.

The worldwide trend is the use of enteral nutrition in all cases when it is possible, if only because its cost is much lower than parenteral, and the efficiency is higher.

For the first time, indications for enteral nutrition were clearly formulated by A. Wretlind & A. Shenkin (1978):

- Enteral nutrition is indicated when the patient cannot eat food (lack of consciousness, swallowing disorders, etc.).

- Enteral nutrition is indicated when the patient should not eat food (acute pancreatitis, gastrointestinal bleeding, etc.).

- Enteral nutrition is indicated when the patient does not want to eat food (anorexia nervosa, infections, etc.).

- Enteral nutrition is indicated when regular nutrition is not adequate to needs (injuries, burns, and catabolism).

Generally the indications for the use of enteral nutrition are:

- Protein-energy deficiency when it is impossible to ensure adequate intake of nutrients by natural oral route.

- Neoplasms, especially localized in the head, neck and stomach.

- Disorders of the central nervous system: coma, cerebrovascular strokes or Parkinson's disease, which result in eating disorders.

- Radiation and chemotherapy for cancer.

- Gastrointestinal tract diseases: Crohn's disease, malabsorption syndrome, short bowel syndrome, chronic pancreatitis, ulcerative colitis, liver and biliary tract diseases.

- Nutrition in the pre - and early postoperative periods.

- Injury, burns, acute poisoning.

- Complications of the postoperative period (fistulas of the gastrointestinal tract, sepsis, failure of sutures of anastomoses).

- Infectious diseases.

- Mental disorders: anorexia nervosa, severe depression.

- Acute and chronic radiation injuries.

Contraindications to Enteral Nutrition

Enteral nutrition is a technique that is intensively studied and applied in an increasingly diverse group of patients. There is a breakdown of stereotypes about mandatory starvation in patients with a field of operations on the gastrointestinal tract, in patients immediately after elimination from a state of shock, and even in patients with pancreatitis. As a result, there is no consensus on the absolute contraindications for enteral nutrition.

Absolute contraindications to enteral nutrition:

- Clinically expressed shock.

- Intestinal ischemia.

- Complete intestinal obstruction (ileus).

- Refusal of the patient or his guardian from conducting enteral nutrition.

- Continued gastrointestinal bleeding.

Relative contraindications to enteral nutrition:

- Partial bowel obstruction.

- Severe, indomitable diarrhea.

- External small intestinal fistulas with detachable more than 500 ml/day.

- Acute pancreatitis and pancreatic cyst. However, there are indications that enteral nutrition is possible even in patients with acute pancreatitis with the distal position of the probe and the use of elemental diets, although there is no consensus on this issue.

- A relative contraindication is the presence of large residual volumes of food (fecal) masses in the intestine (in fact, intestinal paresis).

General Recommendations for Enteral Nutrition

Simple and clear recommendations for enteral nutrition (Jane Standen and David Bihari) are formulated:

- Enteral nutrition should be given as early as possible. Feed through a nasogastric tube if there are no contraindications.

- Enteral nutrition should be started at a rate of 30 ml/hour.

- It is necessary to determine the residual volume as 3 ml/kg.

- It is necessary to aspirate the contents of the probe every 4 hours, and if the residual volume does not exceed 3 ml/hour, then gradually increase the feed rate until the calculated value is reached (25-35 kcal\ kg\day).

- In cases where the residual volume exceeds 3 ml/kg, treatment with prokinetics should be prescribed.

- If, after 24-48 hours, due to the high residual volumes, it is still not possible to adequately feed the patient, then a probe into the ileum should be carried out using the blind method (endoscopically or under the control of an X-ray).

- It should be suggested to the sister who is administering enteral nutrition that if she cannot exercise it properly, it means that she cannot provide the patient with proper care at all.

Nasogastric tube (NG tube)

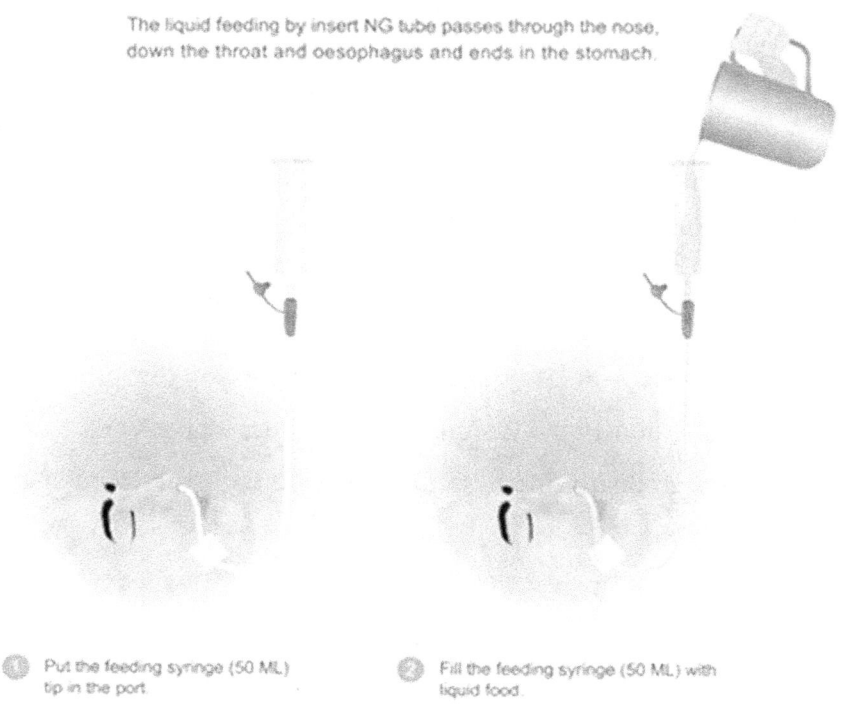

The liquid feeding by insert NG tube passes through the nose, down the throat and oesophagus and ends in the stomach.

1. Put the feeding syringe (50 ML) tip in the port.
2. Fill the feeding syringe (50 ML) with liquid food.

The basis of enteral nutrition is the creation of access to the gastrointestinal tract.

Enteral Nutrition Access Choice

The choice of the point of application of enteral support (stomach, duodenum, jejunum) is determined mainly by the following factors:
- The technical ability to access.
- Risk of aspiration of gastric contents.
- Estimated duration of enteral nutrition.

There are various types of access to the gastrointestinal tract:

- Access at the level of the stomach.

- The simplest and physiological access at the level of the stomach reduces the risk of non-aspiration complications (diarrhea, constipation) and decompression. Still, it requires that the patient be conscious and not have impaired motor function of the stomach.

- Access to the proximal small intestine.

    Access to the proximal sections of the small intestine (duodenum, lean) reduces the risk of aspiration of the gastric contents and nutrient mixture, can be used for impaired consciousness, paresis of the stomach.

- Nasogastric or nasojejunal accesses.

    For short-term enteral nutrition up to 3 weeks, nasogastric or nasojejunal approaches are usually used.

- Access through gastro, duodenostomy.

    When carrying out nutritional support of medium duration (from 3 weeks to 1 year) or long (more than 1 year), it is customary to use percutaneous endoscopic gastro-, duodenostomy or surgical gastro- or jejunostomy.

Types of Probes for Enteral Nutrition

Nasogastric (nasoenteric) and percutaneous probes are used to introduce nutrients. Typically, all probes are radiopaque.

- **Nasogastric and nasoenteric probes.**

    Currently, thin plastic (silicone and polyurethane) probes are mainly used. They can vary somewhat in design: have multi-level openings, bends, be one- or two- or three-lumen, supplied with olives or weighting materials that facilitate their introduction. In the absence of an industrially produced probe, it is possible to use a plastic tube of the appropriate diameter. The use of thick elastic gastric probes is justified only as a temporary access since these probes quickly cause the development of pressure sores.

- **Percutaneous probes.**

    Percutaneous probes are used for accesses created by surgery: pharyngostomy, cervical esophagostomy, gastrostomy, and jejunostomy. The most popular and safe method in recent years is percutaneous endoscopically controlled gastrostomy. It is performed using one-time surgical kits.

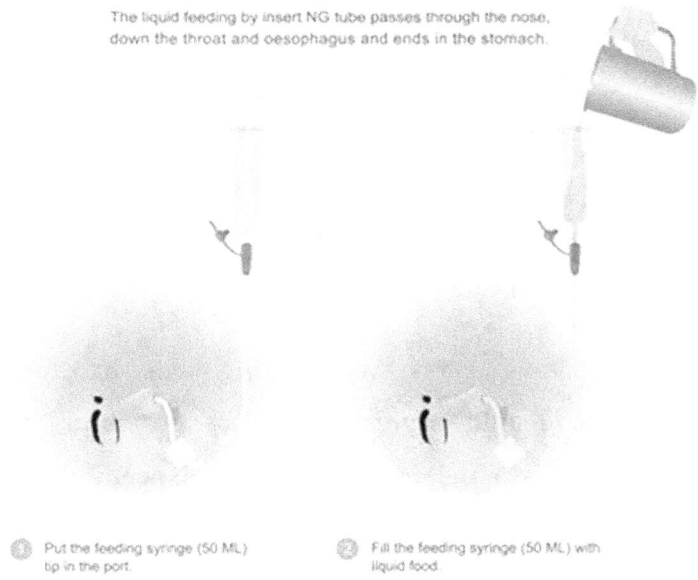

Methods of Introducing Nutrient Mixtures into the Probe

There are two main ways of introducing nutrient mixtures into the probe: passive (gravity-droplet) and active (manual or hardware).

- With the passive method, continuous infusion through a probe is carried out through standard infusion systems (with a destroyed filter) and is regulated by a dispenser.

- The manual method involves the fractional introduction of the nutrient mixture using syringes.

- The most effective is the introduction of mixtures with the help of infusion pumps, which ensure automatic supply of the mixture in a continuous, drip or bolus way.

When to Start Enteral Nutrition

The literature mentions the benefits of "early" parenteral nutrition. Data are presented that in patients with multiple injuries, immediately after stabilization, in the first 6 hours from admission, enteral nutrition was started. Compared with the control group, when nutrition began after 24 hours from admission, a less pronounced violation of the permeability of the intestinal wall and less pronounced multiple organ disorders were noted.

In many resuscitation centers, the following tactics have been adopted: enteral nutrition should begin as early as possible - not only to immediately replenish the patient's energy expenditure, but also to prevent changes in the intestines, which can be achieved by enteral nutrition with relatively small volumes of food.

The theoretical basis for early enteral nutrition

Lack of enteral nutrition leads to:	
Atrophy of the mucosa	It is proved in animal experiments.
Excessive colonization of the small intestine	Enteral nutrition prevents this in lab experiments.
Translocation of bacteria and endotoxins into the portal bloodstream	People have a violation of the permeability of the mucosa during burns, trauma, and critical conditions.

ENTERAL NUTRITION MODES

Nasogastric tube feeding by continuous controlled pump

The feeding tube controlled by electronic pump passes through the nose, throat and oesophagus, continues through the stomach, and ends in the first section of the small intestine.

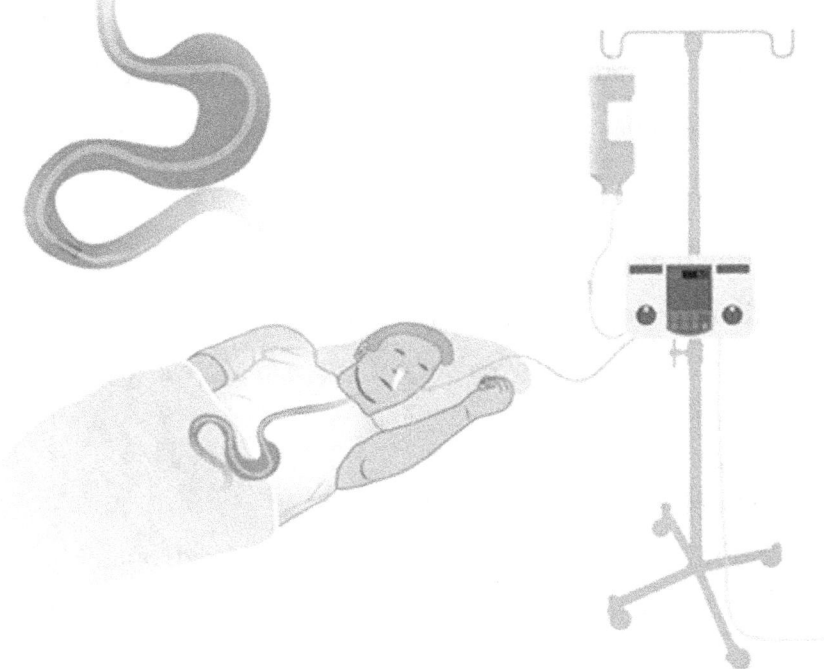

The choice of diet is determined by the condition of the patient, the main and concomitant pathology, and the capabilities of the medical institution. The choice of method, volume, and speed of EP are determined individually for each patient.

The following modes of enteral nutrition are available:

- **Power at a constant speed;**

    Nutrition through a gastric tube begins with isotonic mixtures at a rate of 40-60 ml/h. With good tolerance, the feed rate can be increased by 25 ml/h every 8-12 hours to achieve the desired speed. When feeding through a jejunostomy tube, the initial rate of introduction of the mixture should be 20-30 ml/h, especially in the immediate postoperative period.

    With nausea, vomiting, convulsions, or diarrhea, it is necessary to reduce the rate of administration or concentration of the solution. In this case, simultaneous changes in the feed rate and the concentration of the nutrient mixture should be avoided.

- **Looping food;**

    Continuous drip is gradually "squeezed" to a 10-12 hour night period. Such food, convenient for the patient, can be carried out through a gastrostomy.

- **Periodic or session nutrition;**

    Nutrition with sessions of 4-6 hours is carried out only in the absence of a history of diarrhea, malabsorption syndrome, and operations on the gastrointestinal tract.

- **Bolus nutrition;**

    It imitates a normal meal, therefore, provides a more natural functioning of the gastrointestinal tract. It is carried out only with extraventricular access. The mixture is injected dropwise or with a syringe at a rate of not more than 240 ml in 30 minutes 3-5 times a day. The initial bolus should not exceed 100 ml. With good tolerance, the administered volume is increased daily by 50 ml. Against the background of bolus feeding, diarrhea often develops.

- Usually, if the patient has not received nutrition for several days, a continuous drip of the mixtures is preferable to periodic. Continuous 24-hour nutrition is best used in cases where there are doubts about the safety of the functions of digestion and absorption.

ENTERAL NUTRITION MIXTURES

The choice of a mixture for enteral nutrition depends on many factors: the disease and the general condition of the patient, the presence of violations of the patient's digestive tract, and the required enteral nutrition regimen.

General Requirements for Enteral Mixtures

- The enteral mixture should have a sufficient energy density (at least 1 kcal/ml).

- The enteral mixture should not contain lactose and gluten.

- The enteral mixture should have a low osmolarity (not more than 300-340 mosm/l).

- The enteral mixture should have a low viscosity.

- The enteral mixture should not cause excessive stimulation of intestinal motility.

- The enteral mixture should contain sufficient data on the composition and manufacturer of the nutrient mixture, as well as indications of the presence of genetic modification of nutrients (proteins).

None of the mixtures for complete EP contains a sufficient amount of free water necessary to ensure the patient's daily fluid requirements. The daily fluid requirement is usually estimated at 1 ml per 1 kcal. Most mixtures with an energy value of 1 kcal/ml contain approximately 75% of the required water. Therefore, in the absence of indications for fluid restriction, the amount of additional water consumed by the patient should be approximately 25% of the total amount of food.

At present, mixtures made from natural products or recommended for baby food are not used for enteral nutrition because of their imbalance and inadequacy to the needs of adult patients.

For enteral nutrition, both elemental (modular) formulas and polymer formulas containing proteins, fats, and carbohydrates in proportions characteristic of a normal diet can be used. There are so-called special enteral nutrition formulas developed for various categories of patients.

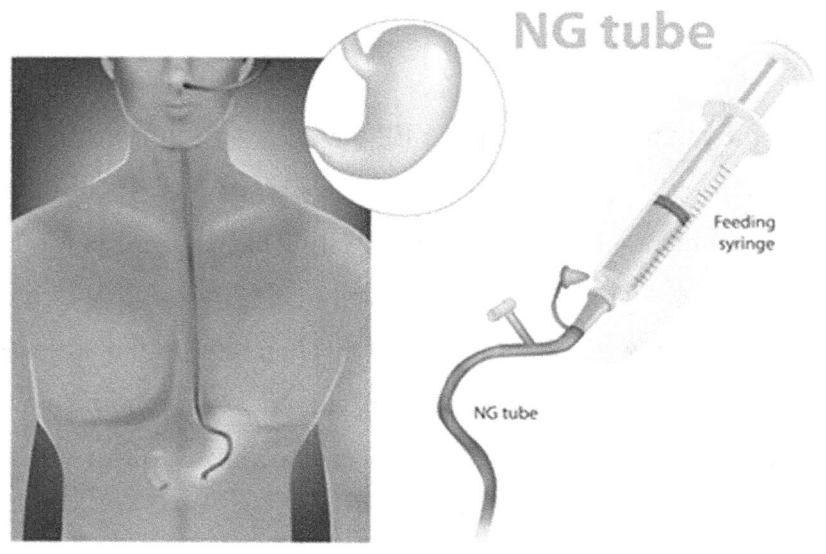

Enteral Nutrition Control

An infusion protocol was developed to improve enteral nutrition and reduce complications. It includes standard medical appointments, sister's responsibilities, provides for the rapid achievement of estimated needs, and limits indications for the cessation of nutrition. This protocol, based on practical recommendations, has significantly improved the enteral nutrition situation in intensive care units.

Enteral Nutrition Protocol In Intensive Care Units

Monitoring of the following indicators is required:

- Clinical data: body temperature, pulse, blood pressure, respiratory rate, flatulence, stool, fluid loss (diuresis, perspiration, by probes).

- Somatometric data: body weight, BMI, shoulder circumference, fold thickness above the triceps, and shoulder muscle circumference.

- Laboratory data: general blood test (hemoglobin, red blood cells, white blood cells, lymphocytes, hematocrit); total blood protein, albumin, transferrin, urea, creatinine, cholesterol, glucose, potassium, sodium, calcium, chloride, AlAT, AsAT, bilirubin, osmolarity; urea nitrogen.

Enteral Nutrition Complications

Prevention of complications is strict adherence to the rules of enteral nutrition.

The high frequency of complications of enteral nutrition is one of the main limiting factors for its widespread use in critical patients. The presence of complications leads to a frequent cessation of enteral nutrition. There are quite objective reasons for such a high frequency of complications of enteral nutrition.

- Enteral nutrition is carried out in a severe category of patients, with damage to all organs and systems of the body, including the gastrointestinal tract.

- Enteral nutrition is necessary only for those patients who already have an intolerance to natural food for various reasons.

- Enteral nutrition is not natural nutrition, but artificial, specially prepared mixtures.

Classification Of Enteral Nutrition Complications

The following types of complications of enteral nutrition are distinguished:

- Infectious complications (aspiration pneumonia, sinusitis, otitis media, wound infection with gastroenterostomies).

- Gastrointestinal complications (diarrhea, constipation, bloating, regurgitation).

- Metabolic complications (hyperglycemia, metabolic alkalosis, hypokalemia, hypophosphatemia).

This classification does not include complications associated with the enteral nutrition technique - self-extraction, migration, and plugging of probes and tubes for nutrition. In addition, a gastrointestinal complication such as regurgitation may coincide with such an infectious complication as aspiration pneumonia, starting with the most frequent and significant.

The literature indicates the frequency of various complications. A wide scatter of data is explained by the fact that there are no unified diagnostic criteria for determining a particular complication, and there is no single protocol for managing complications.

- High residual volumes - 25% -39%.

- Constipation - 15.7%. With prolonged enteral nutrition, the frequency of constipation can increase up to 59%.

- Diarrhea - 14.7% -21% (from 2 to 68%).

- Bloating - 13.2% -18.6%.
- Vomiting - 12.2% -17.8%.
- Regurgitation - 5.5%.
- Aspiration pneumonia - 2%. According to various authors, the frequency of aspiration pneumonia is indicated from 1 to 70 percent.

Residual Volumes, Vomiting, Regurgitation, And Aspiration

The residual volume is the volume of content that remains in the stomach (intestine) during enteral nutrition. The residual volume is used as a criterion of tolerance to nutrition. It depends mainly on the state of motility of the stomach (intestines). In critically ill patients with a traumatic brain injury, on mechanical ventilation receiving sedatives, gastric motility is often reduced. The critical residual volume, upon receipt of which enteral nutrition should be discontinued, is often defined as 200 ml or 3 ml/kg. The presence of residual volume in the stomach in a critical patient is dangerous by the occurrence of vomiting, regurgitation, and aspiration. In the presence of such residual volumes, some authors suggest stopping enteral nutrition and, after 6 hours, try to resume it, while others prefer the appointment of prokinetics.

If it is not possible to establish nutrition within 24-48 hours through the stomach, then it is recommended to install the probe for the pylorus or the tracheal ligament. In this case, the stomach should be drained.

The use of wide probes for nutrition can promote regurgitation due to the impaired function of the esophageal sphincter.

With the development of aspiration pneumonia, mortality is estimated from 41 to 100% and depends on the amount of aspirated volume and the degree of lung tissue involvement. The x-ray picture of aspiration pneumonia is fully manifested during the first 24 hours. If aspiration is diagnosed, it is recommended that as much aspirate be evacuated from the tracheobronchial tree as possible, lavage, debridement bronchoscopy, and decompression of the stomach with a mandatory clarification of the position of the probe. It must be remembered that vomiting and regurgitation can occur during the migration of the probe from the stomach. As maintenance therapy for aspiration pneumonia, mechanical ventilation is performed.

As preventive measures for regurgitation and aspiration, they recommend strict adherence to the protocol, monitoring of residual volumes, correct placement of the probe, and monitoring its position, raising the head of the bed by 35–40°, and avoiding any position.

Diarrhea

Complication is not as dangerous for the patient as aspiration. Diarrhea is a frequent complication of enteral nutrition (from 2 to 68%). Enteral nutrition is suggested to be considered diarrhea as no less than five times loose stools for 24 hours or loose stools with a volume of more than 2000 ml/day. Half-formed stool should not be considered diarrhea, even if its frequency is 6-7 times a day.

The causes of diarrhea are many. Firstly, intestinal infection or intoxication, since enteral nutrition mixtures are a good medium for the growth of microorganisms, and intensive care units are a good supplier of the latter. Diarrhea can cause the introduction of various medications. Many oral suspensions (such as acetaminophen, vitamins, codeine, and other antitussive drugs) contain sorbitol, which can cause diarrhea. Diarrhea also may trigger H2 blockers, antacids containing Mg, digoxin angiotensin-converting enzyme inhibitors, hydralazine, and prokinetics. Antibiotics can also cause diarrhea. Erythromycin, due to its prokinetic properties and all the rest, can cause the development of dysbiosis.

The next group of causes of diarrhea is associated with the characteristics of mixtures for enteral nutrition and the functional state of the gastrointestinal tract. Diarrhea can develop due to the high osmolarity of the mixtures. Normally, the content of the lumen of the gastrointestinal tract is isosmolar to the blood plasma. Mixtures with osmolarity above 400mOsm are believed to cause diarrhea. If the cause of diarrhea is osmolarity, then the transition from a bolus to a constant injection, a decrease in the rate of administration of the mixture, or the use of lower concentrations can stop it.

The cause of diarrhea can also be the lack of dietary fiber in the mixture.

Long-starving patients may develop atrophy of the glands with total enzyme deficiency. In this case, you should switch to semi-element or elemental mixtures and think about enzyme replacement therapy.

In long-starving patients, there is a migration of large intestine bacteria up the gastrointestinal tract with the accumulation of undigested substances, toxins in its lumen, and with the resumption of nutrition and the normal functioning of the gastrointestinal tract, these toxic products are "dumped." There are two conclusions from this: if diarrhea occurs, you should not immediately stop enteral nutrition, since when it resumes, all problems can manifest themselves with renewed vigor.

Do not use drugs that slow down the passage through the gastrointestinal tract (imodium).

It is necessary to prevent dysbiosis. It consists of the timely start of enteral nutrition, the inclusion of dietary fiber in the diet, and the use of biological products.

Bloating

Bloating is defined as visible bloating during a daily examination, tympanitis with percussion, or lack of intestinal murmur. Bloating can be caused by intestinal paresis, and then enteral nutrition is stopped until the causes of paresis are clarified and until it is eliminated. In this case, bloating is combined with high residual volumes and the absence of peristalsis. The causes of paresis are usually external, not directly related to enteral nutrition.

However, sometimes bloating is observed against the background of active peristalsis and with low residual volumes. The cause of increased gas formation may be lactase deficiency, inadequate selection of the mixture (for example, the introduction of natural products into the ileum), and dysbiosis. Management of patients with bloating at low residual volumes has not been developed. Correction of the rate of administration and a change in the qualitative composition of the nutrient mixture, enzyme replacement therapy, treatment of dysbiosis, and the use of symptomatic agents such as activated carbon or espumisan can help. These drugs are not absorbed from the intestinal lumen and do not have any adverse effects on the body. Their use is justified, since defoaming can improve the digestion process and, along with other measures, lead to its full normalization,

Constipation

Constipation is defined as the absence of an independent stool for 2-3 days or the need to use additional funds to obtain it. The frequency of constipation increases significantly with chronic enteral nutrition. Typically, enteral nutrition mixtures are refined products that do not contain the dietary fiber necessary for the normal functioning of the colon. For chronic enteral nutrition, fiber-containing mixtures are recommended. Constipation can also be due to the patient's inactivity and insufficient fluid intake. In fighting constipation, diet correction, the use of laxatives or dietary supplements for food enriched with PV and enemas are recommended.

Metabolic Complications

Most of the metabolic complications are due to the imbalance of the injected mixtures. The following metabolic complications are listed in the literature:

- Hyperglycemia
- Hyperkalemi
- Hypokalemia
- Hypophosphatemia
- Trace deficiencies
- Vitamin deficiencies
- Essential Fatty Acid Deficiencies

Electrolyte abnormalities in resuscitation patients are easily detected with adequate laboratory monitoring. In chronic enteral nutrition, deficiencies of vitamins and minerals may occur. When using balanced mixtures, such complications should not be observed. Hyperglycemia can occur in a severe patient due to the relative insufficiency of the insular apparatus. It is easy to monitor and can be corrected by insulin administration from the outside if necessary.

The literature describes the "renewal syndrome." The "refeeding syndrome" ("refeeding syndrome") is manifested in hypermetabolic or severely malnourished patients with the resumption of nutrition. It is expressed in hypokalemia and hypophosphatemia, which develop due to the increased need for these electrolytes. For the first time, resumption of feeding syndrome was described with intensive feeding of prisoners who returned from World War II. A pathological condition developed with lethargy, diarrhea, weakness, and a variety of electrolyte disorders, sometimes fatal.

Migration, Clogging Of Probes And Tubes

Carrying out nutritional probes for the gatekeeper is a procedure that requires certain skills, time, and technical costs. Therefore, cases of accidental extraction of the probe are always an annoying complication. Their frequency is estimated from 58 to 100%. The reason is most often the patient's self-extraction of the probe due to perceived discomfort, lack of awareness of the importance of the procedure, inadequacy, and impaired consciousness. Repeated placement of the probe is unpleasant not only because of the expenditure of manpower and resources, but also because for some time (sometimes quite long), the enteral nutrition is interrupted. Ways to prevent self-extraction are offered both quite traditional - fixation and sedation of an inadequate patient, and quite original - fixation of the probe using a special "bridle."

It is possible that spending time talking with a patient about the importance of enteral nutrition will save the doctor from the time spent on moving the probe. Irrigation of the oropharynx with a solution of lidocaine or lubrication of the probe with a dicain ointment can temporarily relieve unpleasant sensations. Still, it can also disrupt protective reflexes, increasing the risk of aspiration.

The frequency of complications during the passage of the jejunal tube through the gastrostomy (up to 70%) is rather high - occlusion, dislocation, kink, rupture of the jejunal tube, retrograde migration. Moreover, with chronic enteral nutrition over time, complications associated with the feeding tube come to the fore. Some authors consider the high frequency of self-extraction, probes, and tubes as an argument in favor of a jejunostomy.

Clogging of a correctly and remigration of In intensive care units, the blockage rate of probes is approximately 25%. To prevent clogging of the probes with the nutrient mixture, various schemes exist. One of the standard protocols is flushing the probe every 4 hours with 50 ml of water or after bolus injections. Often, blockage of the probes is associated with the introduction of drugs through them. Some medicines do not have a parenteral analog, when using ready-made suspensions, the frequency of occlusion is slightly lower than when crushing tablets. However, tablet forms are crushed for insertion into the probe. Sublingual, buccal forms should not be fragmented, as well as forms with a complex coating, intended for absorption in various parts of the gastrointestinal tract. Well-dispersed tablets dissolve in at least 10 ml of water. Gelatin capsules can be opened and the contents dissolved in water, or the capsule is completely dissolved in warm water. There are tables of chemical incompatibility of drugs.

Nevertheless, all combinations, including the nutritional formula, cannot be foreseen. Therefore, discrete administration of medications spaced in time, with preliminary and subsequent washing with 50 ml of water, is recommended. The frequency of occlusions when the probe is in the stomach is higher (44%) than when it is in the duodenum (15%), which is associated with the acidity of the contents.

Other Complications

The "others" include complications mainly associated with the technique of enteral nutrition.

With prolonged exposure to the digestive tract, erosion of the nasal mucosa, pharynx, and esophagus can occur. They are more likely when using polyvinyl chloride probes, which become stiff after 7-10 days. Polyurethane and silicone probes can be in the digestive tract for up to 6-8 weeks without the formation of pressure sores. When using a red rubber probe, a pressure sore can occur after 24 hours.

Sinusitis and otitis media often occur in patients with nasogastric tubes and with impaired consciousness. When a diagnosis is made, the probe is removed, saline drops, vasoconstrictors, and antibiotics are prescribed for 3-4 days.

Such complications of blind methods of introducing probes as perforation of the trachea and bronchi, intense pneumothorax, perforation of the mucous membrane of the oropharynx, esophagus, duodenum, and even intracranial migration of the probe are described. This is due to the use of rigid conductors-mandrins for the introduction of thin probes.

There is a possibility of cardiac arrhythmias during manipulations in the area of reflexogenic zones of the oral and nasopharynx.

When using surgical methods to create access for enteral nutrition, a group of corresponding complications also arise. This is pneumoperitoneum, infection around the wound, abdominal abscess, granulomas, bleeding, migration of the food tube along the gastrointestinal tract with the development of intestinal obstruction, etc.

About Sterility With Enteral Nutrition

As one of the advantages of enteral nutrition over parenteral nutrition, the necessity of its sterility is mentioned. However, it must be remembered that, on the one hand, enteral nutrition mixtures are an ideal medium for the reproduction of microorganisms and, on the other hand, in intensive care units, there are all conditions for bacterial aggression. The danger is both the possibility of infection of the patient with microorganisms from the nutrient mixture and poisoning with the resulting endotoxin. It must be taken into account that enteral nutrition is always bypassing the bactericidal barrier of the oropharynx. And as a rule, enteral mixtures are not treated with gastric juice, which has pronounced bactericidal properties, as other factors concomitant with the development of infection, antibiotic therapy is called.

Typical recommendations for the prevention of bacterial contamination are: the use of volumes of a mixture prepared in place of not more than 500 ml. And their use for no more than 8 hours (for sterile factory solutions - 24 hours). In the literature, there are almost no experimentally sound recommendations on the frequency of replacement of probes, bags, droppers. It seems reasonable that for droppers and bags, this should be at least once every 24 hours.

PARENTERAL NUTRITION

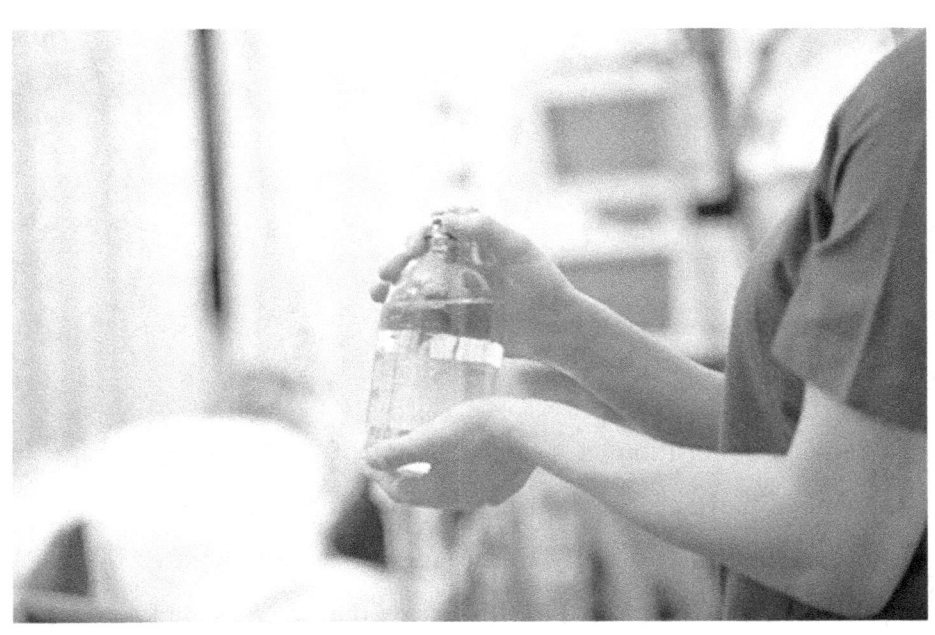

Intravenous feeding

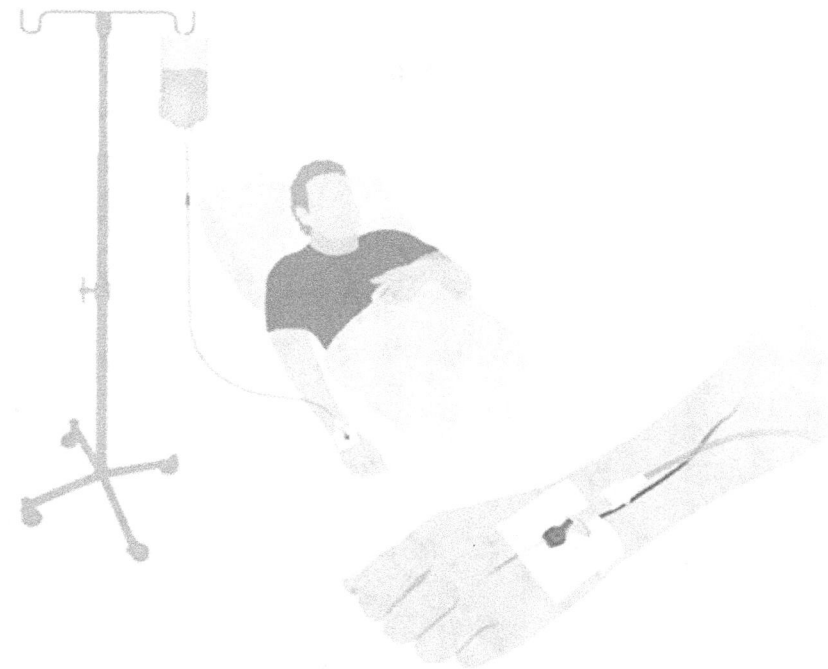

Injection of a solution containing sufficient nutrients in appropriate concentration into the vein.

Parenteral nutrition is a special type of replacement therapy in which nutrients are introduced into the body, to bypass the gastrointestinal tract directly to the internal environment of the body (usually in the vascular bed) to fill energy, plastic costs, and maintain a normal level of metabolic processes. .

The essence of parenteral nutrition is to provide the body with all the substrates necessary for normal functioning involved in the regulation of protein, carbohydrate, fat, water-electrolyte, vitamin metabolism, and acid-base balance.

Classification Of Parenteral Nutrition

- **Complete (total) parenteral nutrition;**

  Full (total) parenteral nutrition provides the entire amount of the daily needs of the body in plastic and energy substrates, as well as maintaining the necessary level of metabolic processes.

- **Incomplete (partial) parenteral nutrition;**

  Incomplete (partial) parenteral nutrition is auxiliary and is aimed at selective replenishment of the deficit of those ingredients, the intake or assimilation of which is not provided by the enteral route. Incomplete parenteral nutrition is considered as additional nutrition if it is used in combination with a tube or oral administration of nutrients.

- **Mixed artificial nutrition;**

  Mixed artificial nutrition is a combination of enteral and parenteral nutrition in cases where none of them is predominant.

The Main Tasks Of Parenteral Nutrition

- Restoration and maintenance of water-electrolyte and acid-base balance.
- Providing the body with energy and plastic substrates.
- Providing the body with all the necessary vitamins, macro- and microelements.

Parenteral Nutrition Concepts

Two main concepts of software have been developed;

- The "American concept," - a hyperalimentation system, according to S. Dudrick (1966) - implies the separate administration of carbohydrate solutions with electrolytes and nitrogen sources.

- The "European concept," - created by A. Wretlind (1964), implies the separate introduction of plastic, carbohydrate, and fatty substrates. Its later version is the "three in one" concept (C. Solassol & H. Joyeux ; 1974), according to which all the necessary nutrition components (amino acids, monosaccharides, fat emulsions, electrolytes, and vitamins) are mixed before administration in a single container under aseptic conditions.

- In recent years, many countries have begun to apply the all-in-one parenteral nutrition methodology using 3-liter containers to mix all the ingredients in one plastic bag. If it is impossible to mix three-in-one solutions, infusion of plastic and energy substrates should be carried out in parallel (preferably through a V-shaped adapter).

- In recent years, ready-made mixtures of amino acids and fat emulsions have been produced. The advantages of this method are minimized manipulations with containers containing nutrients, their infection is reduced, and the risk of hyperglycemia and hyperosmolar non-ketone coma is reduced. Disadvantages: gluing fatty particles and the formation of large globules that could be dangerous for the patient, the problem of catheter occlusion has not been solved, it is not known how long this mixture can safely be in the refrigerator.

Basic Principles Of Parenteral Nutrition

- Timely start of parenteral nutrition.

- The optimal timing of parenteral nutrition (until restoration of normal trophic status).

- Adequacy (balance) of parenteral nutrition in terms of the amount of nutrients introduced and the degree of their absorption.

Rules For Parenteral Nutrition

- Nutrients should be administered in a form adequate to the metabolic needs of the cells, that is, similar to the intake of nutrients into the bloodstream after passing the enteric barrier. Accordingly: proteins in the form of amino acids, fats - fat emulsions, carbohydrates - monosaccharides.

- Strict adherence to the appropriate rate of introduction of nutrient substrates is necessary.

- Plastic and energy substrates must be introduced simultaneously. Be sure to use all the essential nutrients.

- Infusion of highly osmolar solutions (especially exceeding 900 mosmol/l) should be carried out only in the central veins.

- Parenteral nutrition infusion systems change every 24 hours.

- When conducting a full parenteral nutrition, the inclusion of glucose concentrates in the mixture is mandatory.

- The fluid requirement for a stable patient is 1 ml/kcal or 30 ml/kg body weight. In pathological conditions, the need for water increases.

Indications For Parenteral Nutrition

When conducting parenteral nutrition, it is important to consider that in the conditions of termination or restriction of the intake of nutrients by the exogenous route, the most important adaptive mechanism comes into play: the expenditure of mobile reserves of carbohydrates, body fats, and intensive protein breakdown to amino acids with their subsequent conversion into carbohydrates. Such metabolic activity, being at first expedient, designed to ensure vital activity, subsequently very negatively affects the course of all life processes. Therefore, it is advisable to cover the needs of the body not due to the breakdown of their own tissues, but due to exogenous intake of nutrients.

The main objective criterion for the use of parenteral nutrition is a pronounced negative nitrogen balance, which cannot be corrected by the enteral route. The average daily nitrogen loss in resuscitation patients is from 15 to 32 g, which corresponds to a loss of 94-200 g of tissue protein or 375-800 g of muscle tissue.

The main indications for parenteral nutrition can be divided into several groups:

- The impossibility of oral or enteral food intake for at least 7 days in a stable patient, or in a shorter time in a depleted patient (this group of indications is usually associated with impaired gastrointestinal function).

- Severe hypermetabolism or significant loss of protein, when only enteral nutrition is not allowed to cope with nutrient deficiency (a classic example is a burn disease).

- The need for a temporary exclusion of intestinal digestion "bowel rest" (for example, with ulcerative colitis).

Indications For Parenteral Nutrition

Full parenteral nutrition is indicated in all cases when it is impossible to take food naturally or through a tube, which is accompanied by increased catabolic and inhibition of anabolic processes, as well as a negative nitrogen balance:

- In the preoperative period in patients with symptoms of complete or partial starvation in diseases of the gastrointestinal tract in cases of functional or organic lesions of it with digestive disorders and resorption.

- In the postoperative period after extensive operations on the organs of the abdominal cavity or its complicated course (failure of anastomoses, fistulas, peritonitis, sepsis).

- In the post-traumatic period (severe burns, multiple injuries).
- With increased protein breakdown or a violation of its synthesis (hyperthermia, insufficiency of the liver, kidneys, etc.).
- Resuscitation patients, when the patient does not regain consciousness for a long time or the gastrointestinal tract activity is sharply disturbed (CNS lesions, tetanus, acute poisoning, coma, etc.).
- In infectious diseases (cholera, dysentery).
- With neuropsychic diseases in cases of anorexia, vomiting, refusal of food.

Contraindications For Parenteral Nutrition
Absolute Contraindications

- The period of shock, hypovolemia, electrolyte disturbances.
- Possibility of adequate enteral and oral nutrition.
- Allergic reactions to parenteral nutrition components.
- Failure of the patient (or his guardian).
- Cases in which parenteral nutrition does not improve the prognosis of the disease.

In some of these situations, the elements of parenteral nutrition can be used during complex intensive care of patients.

Contraindications to the Use of Certain Drugs

Contraindications to the use of certain drugs for parenteral nutrition determine pathological changes in the body due to underlying and concomitant diseases.

- In the case of hepatic or renal failure, amino acid mixtures and fat emulsions are contraindicated.

- With hyperlipidemia, lipoid nephrosis, signs of post-traumatic fat embolism, acute myocardial infarction, cerebral edema, diabetes mellitus, fat emulsions are contraindicated in the first 5-6 days of the post-resuscitation period and in violation of the coagulating properties of the blood.

- Caution must be exercised in patients with allergic diseases.

Providing Parenteral Nutrition
Infusion Technology

The main method of parenteral nutrition is the introduction of energy, plastic substrates, and other ingredients into the vascular bed: into peripheral veins, into the central veins, into the recanalized umbilical vein, through shunts, and intra-arterially.

When conducting parenteral nutrition, infusion pumps and electronic droplet regulators are used. The infusion should be carried out within 24 hours at a certain speed, but not more than 30-40 drops per minute. At this rate of administration, the enzyme systems are not overloaded with nitrogen-containing substances.

Access

The following access options are currently used:

- Through a peripheral vein (using a cannula or catheter), it is usually used when initializing parenteral nutrition for up to 1 day or with additional parenteral nutrition.

- Through the central vein using temporary central catheters. Among the central veins, subclavian vein is preferred. Less commonly used are the internal jugular and femoral vein.

- Through the central vein using permanent central catheters.

- Through alternative vascular accesses and extravascular accesses (e.g., peritoneal cavity).

Parenteral Nutrition

- Round-the-clock introduction of nutrient media.

- Prolonged infusion (within 18–20 hours).

- Cyclic regimen (infusion for 8-12 hours).

Preparations For Parenteral Nutrition

Basic Requirements for Parenteral Nutrition

Based on the principles of parenteral nutrition, funds for parenteral nutrition should meet several basic requirements:

- To have a nutritious effect, that is, to have in its composition all the substances necessary for the body in a sufficient amount and proper proportions with each other.

- Replenish the body with fluid, as many conditions are accompanied by dehydration.

- It is highly desirable to have detoxification and stimulating effects on the drugs used.

- It is desirable to substitute and anti-shock effect of the applied means.

- It is necessary to verify the safety of the means used.

- An important component is the ease of use.

Characteristics Of Parenteral Nutrition

For the proper use of nutrient solutions for parenteral nutrition, it is necessary to evaluate some of their characteristics:

- The osmolarity of solutions for parenteral nutrition.

- The energy value of solutions.

- The limits of maximum infusions are the rate or rate of infusion.
- When planning parenteral nutrition, the necessary doses of energy substrates, minerals, and vitamins are calculated based on their daily needs and energy consumption.

Parenteral Nutrition Components

The main components of parenteral nutrition are usually divided into two groups: energy donors (carbohydrate solutions - monosaccharides and alcohols and fat emulsions) and plastic material donors (solutions of amino acids). Means for parenteral nutrition consist of the following components:

- Carbohydrates and alcohols are the main sources of energy for parenteral nutrition.
- Sorbitol (20%) and xylitol are used as additional energy sources with glucose and fat emulsions.
- Fats are the most effective energy substrate. They are introduced in the form of fat emulsions.
- Proteins are the most important component for building tissues, blood, synthesis of proteogormones, and enzymes.
- Saline solutions: simple and complex, are introduced to normalize the water-electrolyte and acid-base balance.
- Vitamins, minerals, anabolic hormones are also included in the complex of parenteral nutrition.

Assessment Of The Patient's Condition If Parenteral Nutrition Is Necessary

When conducting parenteral nutrition, it is necessary to take into account the individual characteristics of the patient, the nature of the disease, metabolism, as well as the energy needs of the body.

- Evaluation of nutrition and monitoring the adequacy of parenteral nutrition;

The goal is to determine the type and extent of malnutrition, as well as the need for nutritional support.

The nutritional status in recent years is assessed based on the definition of trophic or trophological status, which is considered as an indicator of physical development and health. Trophic insufficiency is established based on an anamnesis, somatometric, laboratory, clinical, and functional indicators.

- Somatometric indicators; these are the most affordable and include the measurement of body weight, shoulder circumference, thickness of the skin-fat fold, and the calculation of body mass index.

- Laboratory tests;

Serum albumin; when it decreases below 35g/l, the number of complications increases by 4 times, mortality by 6 times.

Serum transferrin; its decrease indicates the depletion of visceral protein (normal 2g/l or more).

Excretion of creatinine, urea, 3-methylhistidine (3-MG) with urine; A decrease in creatinine and 3-MG excreted in the urine indicates a muscle protein deficiency. The ratio of 3-MG/creatinine reflects the direction of metabolic processes in the direction of anabolism or catabolism and the effectiveness of parenteral nutrition for the correction of protein deficiency (excretion in the urine of 4.2 µM 3-MG corresponds to the breakdown of 1g of muscle protein).

Monitoring the concentration of glucose in the blood and urine: the appearance of sugar in the urine and an increase in the concentration of glucose in the blood more than 2 g/l require not so much an increase in the dose of insulin as a decrease in the amount of glucose administered.

- Clinical and functional indicators: reduced tissue turgor, the presence of cracks, edema, etc.

The Energy Needs Of The Body
Monitoring Parenteral Nutrition

The parameters for monitoring homeostasis indicators during a full parenteral nutrition were determined in Amsterdam in 1981.

Monitoring is carried out over the state of metabolism, the presence of infectious complications, and nutritional efficiency. Indicators such as body temperature, heart rate, blood pressure, and respiratory rate are determined in patients daily. The determination of the main laboratory parameters in unstable patients is mainly carried out 1-3 times a day, with meals in the pre- and postoperative period 1-3 times a week, with long-term parenteral nutrition - 1 time per week.

Particular importance is attached to indicators characterizing the adequacy of nutrition - protein (urea nitrogen, serum albumin, and prothrombin time), carbohydrate (blood glucose and urine glucose), and lipid (serum triglycerides).

Complications Of Parenteral Nutrition

There are technical, metabolic, organopathological and septic complications. Prevention of all types of complications is the strict observance of all the rules for the introduction of parenteral solutions and monitoring of homeostasis.

Technical Complications

Technical complications are usually associated with creating access to the vascular system: pneumothorax and hydrothorax, embolism, tearing of the catheter-carrying vein, and others. Their prevention is associated with compliance with the installation and operation of the intravenous feeding tract.

On the border of technical and infectious complications are thrombosis (and thrombophlebitis) of the catheter, central and peripheral veins.

METABOLIC COMPLICATIONS

Organopathological Complications

Respiratory complications - hypercapnia with the introduction of excess monosaccharides, especially in the form of concentrated solutions. In depleted patients, with the introduction of the mixture, an increase in the formation of CO_2 may not be accompanied by an increase in the minute volume of respiration, which leads to respiratory disorders.

The introduction of carbohydrate solutions leads to the activation of liponeogenesis with the formation of fatty liver. With the development of steatohepatitis, it is necessary to reduce the total calorie intake or increase the proportion of fat emulsion.

Rehabilitation syndrome - with the forced use of monosaccharides, against the background of anabolism, potassium, magnesium, and phosphate move into the intracellular space.

With excessive protein intake, ventilation of patients with chronic obstructive pulmonary diseases is stimulated, and pulmonary dysfunction may develop.

In cases where standard amino acid solutions are administered to patients with impaired liver function, a deterioration in the state of mind associated with hepatic encephalopathy can be expected.

With prolonged, mainly complete parenteral nutrition, some organopathological complications arise; diseases of the gallbladder associated with changes in the composition of bile and a decrease in contractile activity of the gallbladder; bone disorders caused by a change in the metabolism of vitamin D.

Septic Complications

Septic complications are most often associated with a violation of the rules of asepsis and antiseptics. Infectious complications are catheter infections with the development of angiogenic sepsis.

Prevention of infectious complications consists of observing the rules of asepsis, caring for catheters, using silicone venous catheters, and protective films.

Complications Associated With The Introduction Of Fat Emulsions

The most common violation with the introduction of fat emulsions is the development of hypertriglyceridemia, caused by the high rate of administration of emulsions and impaired lipid metabolism. To prevent hypertriglyceridemia, heparin is added at a rate of 1–10 PIECES per 1 ml of emulsion, which improves triglyceride clearance through the mechanism of lipoprotein lipase stimulation.

The difference between early and late complications associated with the introduction of fat emulsions;

- Early complications are caused by acute reactions to infusion (shortness of breath, cyanosis, allergies, nausea, vomiting, headache, lower back pain, fever, dizziness, sweating, inflammation at the site of infusion), and hypersensitivity reactions.

- Late complications (fat overload syndrome) are manifested by hepatomegaly with cholestasis and hematological disorders (splenomegaly, thrombocyte, and leukopenia).

ENTERAL OR PARENTERAL NUTRITION?

Nutritional support, that is, providing the body with the necessary amount of energy and building substrates for its life, is an absolutely essential part of intensive care. Exercising it through the gastrointestinal tract is the best and safest method. If there is no significant loss of fluid through the intestines, paresis, and massive gastroduodenal bleeding, then, in any case, you should check how the digestive tract is suitable for enteral nutrition.

Alternative - parenteral nutrition is used only if it is impossible to carry out enteral (intestinal fistula with significant discharge, short bowel syndrome or malabsorption, intestinal obstruction, etc.).

Parenteral nutrition is several times more expensive than enteral. During its implementation, strict adherence to the sterility and speed of introduction of the ingredients is required, which is associated with certain technical difficulties. Parenteral nutrition provides a sufficient number of complications. There is evidence that parenteral nutrition can inhibit your own immunity.

In any case, during complete parenteral nutrition, intestinal atrophy occurs - atrophy from inactivity. Atrophy of the mucosa leads to ulceration. Atrophy of the secreting glands leads to subsequent enzymatic deficiency, stagnation of bile, uncontrolled growth, and change in the composition of intestinal microflora, and atrophy of lymphoid tissue associated with the intestine.

Enteral nutrition is more physiological. It does not require sterility. Enteral nutritional mixtures contain all the necessary components. Calculation of potency in enteral nutrition and the procedure for its implementation are much simpler than with parenteral nutrition. Enteral nutrition helps maintain the gastrointestinal tract in a normal physiological state and prevent many complications that arise in critically ill patients. Enteral nutrition leads to improved blood circulation in the intestine and contributes to the normal healing of anastomoses after operations on the intestine. Thus, in all cases, when it is possible, the choice of the method of nutritional support should be inclined towards enteral nutrition.

AUTHOR'S PRESENTATION

Dr. Amin Gasmi is a physiologist and orthomolecular nutritionist. He is currently the president of the Francophone Society of Nutritherapy and Applied Nutrigenetics. He is also the founder and managing editor of the International Journal of Integrative Physiology and Nutritional Sciences. He is a member of several international scientific organizations such as the International Society of Immunonutrition and the International Society of Orthomolecular Medicine. Dr. Gasmi has a multidisciplinary background and had the opportunity to work on several fields such as nutrition sciences, micronutrition, genetics, exercise physiology, applied psychology, physical therapy, physical training, and biochemistry. He has a triple competence of clinician through patients' and athletes' nutritional and physiological care, of scientist through his high quality published books and articles, and of professional trainer through the trainings and lectures he gives to medical doctors, health, and sports professionals.

REFERENCES

Chowdary, K. V., & Reddy, P. N. (2010). Parenteral nutrition: Revisited. *Indian journal of anaesthesia*, *54*(2), 95–103. https://doi.org/10.4103/0019-5049.63637

Cotogni P. (2017). Management of parenteral nutrition in critically ill patients. *World journal of critical care medicine*, *6*(1), 13–20. https://doi.org/10.5492/wjccm.v6.i1.13

Dudrick S.J. (2009) History of Parenteral Nutrition, *Journal of the American College of Nutrition*, 28:3, 243-251, DOI: 10.1080/07315724.2009.10719778

Hartl, W. H., Jauch, K. W., Parhofer, K., Rittler, P., & Working group for developing the guidelines for parenteral nutrition of The German Association for Nutritional Medicine (2009). Complications and monitoring - Guidelines on Parenteral Nutrition, Chapter 11. *German medical science: GMS e-journal*, *7*, Doc17. https://doi.org/10.3205/000076

Lappas, B. M., Patel, D., Kumpf, V., Adams, D. W., & Seidner, D. L. (2018). Parenteral Nutrition: Indications, Access, and Complications. *Gastroenterology clinics of North America*, *47*(1), 39–59. https://doi.org/10.1016/j.gtc.2017.10.001

Maudar K. K. (1995). TOTAL PARENTERAL NUTRITION. *Medical journal, Armed Forces India*, *51*(2), 122–126. https://doi.org/10.1016/S0377-1237(17)30942-5

Nguyen D. L. (2017). Guidance for supplemental enteral nutrition across patient populations. *The American journal of managed care*, *23*(12 Suppl), S210–S219.

Seres, D. S., Valcarcel, M., & Guillaume, A. (2013). Advantages of enteral nutrition over parenteral nutrition. *Therapeutic advances in gastroenterology*, *6*(2), 157–167.https://doi.org/10.1177/1756283X12467564

Seron-Arbeloa, C., Zamora-Elson, M., Labarta-Monzon, L., & Mallor-Bonet, T. (2013). Enteral nutrition in critical care. *Journal of clinical medicine research*, *5*(1), 1–11. https://doi.org/10.4021/jocmr1210w

Shenkin, A., Wretlind, A. (1978) Parenteral nutrition. *World Rev Nutr Diet*, 28:1

Solassol C, Joyeux H, Etco L, Pujol H, Romieu C. (1974) New techniques for long-term intravenous feeding: an artificial gut in 75 patients. *Ann Surg*, 179(4):519-522

Wretlind A. (1964) The pharmacological basis for the use of fat emulsions in intravenous nutrition. *Acta Chir Scand Suppl*, 325:31+

www.ingramcontent.com/pod-product-compliance
Lightning Source LLC
Chambersburg PA
CBHW071147240526
45465CB00024BA/1842